1

Table of Contents

Introduction

Understanding Graves' Disease

Graves' disease is an autoimmune disorder that causes hyperthyroidism, a condition in which the thyroid gland produces excessive amounts of thyroid hormone. This can lead to a variety of symptoms and complications if not properly managed. Understanding the basics of Graves' disease is crucial for those affected and their loved ones.

What is Graves' Disease?

Graves' disease is the most common cause of hyperthyroidism. It occurs when the body's immune system mistakenly attacks the thyroid gland, a small butterfly-shaped gland located at the base of the neck. This immune system malfunction causes the thyroid gland to produce too much thyroid hormone, leading to a range of symptoms.

Symptoms of Graves' Disease

Graves' disease can cause a variety of symptoms, including:

Increased heart rate or palpitations

Unexplained weight loss

Fatigue or muscle weakness

Tremors (shaking hands or fingers)

Increased sensitivity to heat

Increased appetite

Irritability or nervousness

Difficulty sleeping

More frequent bowel movements

Enlarged thyroid gland (goiter)

Bulging eyes (exophthalmos)

Diagnosis and Treatment

Diagnosing Graves' disease typically involves a combination of physical exams, blood tests to measure thyroid hormone levels, and imaging tests such as a thyroid ultrasound or radioactive iodine uptake test. Once diagnosed, treatment options may include medications to regulate thyroid hormone levels, radioactive iodine therapy to reduce thyroid activity, or surgery to remove part or all of the thyroid gland.

The Role of Diet in Graves' Disease

While diet alone cannot cure Graves' disease, it can play a supportive role in managing symptoms and promoting overall health. A diet for Graves' disease typically focuses on nutrient-dense foods, limiting iodine-rich foods, and managing goitrogenic foods that can interfere with thyroid function. Working with a healthcare provider or dietitian to develop a personalized diet plan is recommeThe Role of Diet in Managing Graves' Disease

Diet plays a crucial role in managing Graves' disease, an autoimmune disorder that causes hyperthyroidism. While diet alone cannot cure the condition, it can help alleviate symptoms, support thyroid function, and promote overall well-being. Here's how diet can be beneficial for individuals with Graves' disease:

1. Nutrient-Dense Foods: Consuming a diet rich in vitamins, minerals, and antioxidants can support overall health and help manage symptoms. Focus on incorporating a variety of fruits, vegetables, whole grains, and lean proteins into your meals.

2. Iodine Regulation: Excessive iodine intake can exacerbate hyperthyroidism in individuals with Graves' disease. Avoiding or limiting foods high in iodine, such as iodized salt, seafood, and seaweed, can help regulate thyroid function.

3. Goitrogenic Foods: Some foods contain compounds called goitrogens, which can interfere with thyroid function. Cooking these foods can reduce their goitrogenic effects. Examples include broccoli, cabbage, Brussels sprouts, and kale.

4. Selenium Supplementation: Selenium is a mineral that may help reduce inflammation in the thyroid gland. Including selenium-rich foods in

your diet, such as Brazil nuts, sunflower seeds, fish, and eggs, can be beneficial.

5. Balanced Meals: Eating regular, balanced meals can help stabilize blood sugar levels and support energy levels throughout the day. Aim for a mix of carbohydrates, protein, and healthy fats at each meal.

6. Hydration: Staying well-hydrated is important for overall health. Water helps regulate body temperature, supports digestion, and can help prevent dehydration, which can worsen symptoms of hyperthyroidism.

7. Avoid Stimulants: Stimulants like caffeine and alcohol can exacerbate symptoms such as anxiety, palpitations, and insomnia. Limiting or avoiding these substances may help manage these symptoms.

8. Consult a Healthcare Provider: It's important to work with a healthcare provider or registered dietitian to develop a personalized diet plan that meets your individual needs and complements your medical treatment.

Chapter 1: Breakfast Delights

- Energizing Oatmeal Bowl

1. Apple Cinnamon Oatmeal Bowl

- Ingredients:

- 1/2 cup rolled oats

- 1 cup almond milk

- 1 small apple, diced

- 1/2 teaspoon cinnamon

- 1 tablespoon honey or maple syrup

- Method:

1. In a small saucepan, combine oats and almond milk.

2. Bring to a simmer over medium heat, stirring occasionally.

3. Add diced apple and cinnamon, and cook for another 5 minutes.

4. Sweeten with honey or maple syrup, and serve warm.

2. Banana Nut Oatmeal Bowl

- Ingredients:

- 1/2 cup rolled oats

- 1 cup water or milk of choice

- 1 ripe banana, mashed

- 2 tablespoons chopped nuts (e.g., almonds, walnuts)

- 1 tablespoon honey or maple syrup

- Method:

1. Cook oats in water or milk according to package instructions.

2. Stir in mashed banana and chopped nuts.

3. Sweeten with honey or maple syrup, and enjoy.

3. Berry Blast Oatmeal Bowl

- Ingredients:

- 1/2 cup rolled oats

- 1 cup water or milk of choice

- 1/2 cup mixed berries (e.g., strawberries, blueberries, raspberries)

- 1 tablespoon chia seeds

- 1 tablespoon honey or maple syrup

- Method:

1. Cook oats in water or milk according to package instructions.

2. Stir in mixed berries and chia seeds.

3. Sweeten with honey or maple syrup, and serve.

4. Peanut Butter Banana Oatmeal Bowl

- Ingredients:

- 1/2 cup rolled oats

- 1 cup almond milk

- 1 banana, sliced

- 1 tablespoon peanut butter

- 1 tablespoon honey or maple syrup

- Method:

1. In a small saucepan, combine oats and almond milk.

2. Bring to a simmer over medium heat, stirring occasionally.

3. Add sliced banana and peanut butter, and cook for another 5 minutes.

4. Sweeten with honey or maple syrup, and serve warm.

5. Almond Joy Oatmeal Bowl

• Ingredients:

• 1/2 cup rolled oats

• 1 cup coconut milk

• 2 tablespoons shredded coconut

• 1 tablespoon cocoa powder

• 1 tablespoon honey or maple syrup

• Method:

1. Cook oats in coconut milk according to package instructions.

2. Stir in shredded coconut and cocoa powder.

3. Sweeten with honey or maple syrup, and enjoy.

6. Pumpkin Pie Oatmeal Bowl

- Ingredients:

- 1/2 cup rolled oats

- 1 cup almond milk

- 1/4 cup pumpkin puree

- 1/2 teaspoon pumpkin pie spice

- 1 tablespoon honey or maple syrup

- Method:

1. In a small saucepan, combine oats and almond milk.

2. Bring to a simmer over medium heat, stirring occasionally.

3. Add pumpkin puree and pumpkin pie spice, and cook for another 5 minutes.

4. Sweeten with honey or maple syrup, and serve warm.

7. Tropical Paradise Oatmeal Bowl

- Ingredients:

- 1/2 cup rolled oats

- 1 cup coconut milk

- 1/2 banana, sliced

- 1/4 cup chopped pineapple

- 1 tablespoon shredded coconut

- Method:

1. Cook oats in coconut milk according to package instructions.

2. Stir in sliced banana, chopped pineapple, and shredded coconut.

3. Serve warm and enjoy the tropical flavors.

8. Blueberry Almond Oatmeal Bowl

- Ingredients:

- 1/2 cup rolled oats

- 1 cup almond milk

- 1/2 cup blueberries

- 2 tablespoons sliced almonds

- 1 tablespoon honey or maple syrup

- Method:

1. In a small saucepan, combine oats and almond milk.

2. Bring to a simmer over medium heat, stirring occasionally.

3. Add blueberries and sliced almonds, and cook for another 5 minutes.

4. Sweeten with honey or maple syrup, and serve warm.

9. Chocolate Banana Oatmeal Bowl

- Ingredients:

- 1/2 cup rolled oats

- 1 cup almond milk

- 1 banana, sliced

- 1 tablespoon cocoa powder

- 1 tablespoon honey or maple syrup

- Method:

1. In a small saucepan, combine oats and almond milk.

2. Bring to a simmer over medium heat, stirring occasionally.

3. Add sliced banana and cocoa powder, and cook for another 5 minutes.

4. Sweeten with honey or maple syrup, and enjoy the chocolatey goodness.

10. Coconut Chia Oatmeal Bowl

- Ingredients:

- 1/2 cup rolled oats

- 1 cup coconut milk

- 1 tablespoon chia seeds

- 2 tablespoons shredded coconut

- 1 tablespoon honey or maple syrup

- Method:

1. Cook oats in coconut milk according to package instructions.

2. Stir in chia seeds and shredded coconut.

3. Sweeten with honey or maple syrup, and serve warm.

- Avocado Toast with a Twist

1. Avocado and Strawberry Balsamic Toast

Ingredients:

- 1 ripe avocado

- 4 slices of whole grain bread

- 1 cup fresh strawberries, sliced

- Balsamic glaze

- Salt and pepper to taste

Instructions:

1. Toast the bread slices until golden brown.

2. Mash the ripe avocado in a bowl and season with salt and pepper.

3. Spread the mashed avocado evenly on each slice of toast.

4. Top the avocado with sliced strawberries.

5. Drizzle with balsamic glaze.

6. Serve immediately and enjoy!

2. Spicy Avocado and Egg Toast

Ingredients:

• 1 ripe avocado

• 4 slices of whole grain bread

• 4 eggs

• Hot sauce

• Salt and pepper to taste

• Optional: sliced jalapeños for extra heat

Instructions:

1. Toast the bread slices until golden brown.

2. Mash the ripe avocado in a bowl and season with salt and pepper.

3. Spread the mashed avocado evenly on each slice of toast.

4. Cook the eggs to your liking (fried, scrambled, or poached).

5. Place one cooked egg on each slice of toast.

6. Drizzle with hot sauce and add sliced jalapeños if desired.

7. Serve immediately and enjoy!

3. Avocado and Smoked Salmon Toast

Ingredients:

• 1 ripe avocado

• 4 slices of whole grain bread

• 4 oz smoked salmon

• Fresh dill, chopped

• Lemon juice

• Salt and pepper to taste

Instructions:

1. Toast the bread slices until golden brown.

2. Mash the ripe avocado in a bowl and season with salt, pepper, and a squeeze of lemon juice.

3. Spread the mashed avocado evenly on each slice of toast.

4. Top each slice with smoked salmon.

5. Sprinkle with fresh chopped dill.

6. Serve immediately and enjoy!

4. Avocado and Black Bean Toast

Ingredients:

- 1 ripe avocado

- 4 slices of whole grain bread

- 1 can black beans, drained and rinsed

- 1/2 red onion, diced

- 1/2 red bell pepper, diced

- Cilantro, chopped

- Lime juice

- Salt and pepper to taste

Instructions:

1. Toast the bread slices until golden brown.

2. Mash the ripe avocado in a bowl and season with salt, pepper, and a squeeze of lime juice.

3. In a separate bowl, mix the black beans, diced red onion, diced red bell pepper, and chopped cilantro.

4. Spread the mashed avocado evenly on each slice of toast.

5. Top with the black bean mixture.

6. Serve immediately and enjoy!

5. Avocado and Pesto Toast

Ingredients:

- 1 ripe avocado

- 4 slices of whole grain bread

- 1/4 cup store-bought or homemade pesto

- Cherry tomatoes, halved

• Fresh basil leaves

• Salt and pepper to taste

Instructions:

1. Toast the bread slices until golden brown.

2. Mash the ripe avocado in a bowl and season with salt and pepper.

3. Spread the mashed avocado evenly on each slice of toast.

4. Spread a thin layer of pesto over the avocado.

5. Top with halved cherry tomatoes and fresh basil leaves.

6. Serve immediately and enjoy!

These avocado toast variations are not only delicious but also packed with nutrients, making them a healthy and satisfying meal option. Enjoy experimenting with different flavors and ingredients to find your favorite combination!

Chapter 2: Nourishing Soups and Salads

Roasted Vegetable Soup

1. Classic Roasted Vegetables

Ingredients:

- 1 medium zucchini, sliced
- 1 medium yellow squash, sliced
- 1 red bell pepper, seeded and sliced
- 1 yellow bell pepper, seeded and sliced
- 1 red onion, sliced
- 2 tablespoons olive oil
- 2 cloves garlic, minced
- 1 teaspoon dried thyme
- Salt and pepper, to taste

Instructions:

10. Preheat the oven to 400°F (200°C) and line a baking sheet with parchment paper.

11. In a large bowl, combine the zucchini, yellow squash, bell peppers, and onion.

12. Drizzle with olive oil and sprinkle with garlic, thyme, salt, and pepper. Toss to coat evenly.

13. Spread the vegetables in a single layer on the prepared baking sheet.

14. Roast in the preheated oven for 25-30 minutes, or until the vegetables are tender and lightly browned, stirring halfway through cooking.

2. Balsamic Roasted Vegetables

Ingredients:

• 1 large sweet potato, peeled and cubed

• 2 carrots, peeled and sliced

• 1 red onion, sliced

• 1 red bell pepper, seeded and sliced

• 2 tablespoons olive oil

• 2 tablespoons balsamic vinegar

• 1 teaspoon dried rosemary

• Salt and pepper, to taste

Instructions:

8. Preheat the oven to 400°F (200°C) and line a baking sheet with parchment paper.

9. In a large bowl, combine the sweet potato, carrots, onion, and bell pepper.

10. Drizzle with olive oil and balsamic vinegar. Sprinkle with rosemary, salt, and pepper. Toss to coat evenly.

11. Spread the vegetables in a single layer on the prepared baking sheet.

12. Roast in the preheated oven for 25-30 minutes, or until the vegetables are tender and caramelized, stirring halfway through cooking.

3. Curry Roasted Vegetables

Ingredients:

• 1 small head cauliflower, cut into florets

• 2 medium carrots, peeled and sliced

• 1 red onion, sliced

- 2 tablespoons olive oil

- 1 tablespoon curry powder

- 1 teaspoon ground cumin

- 1/2 teaspoon turmeric

- Salt and pepper, to taste

Instructions:

8. Preheat the oven to 400°F (200°C) and line a baking sheet with parchment paper.

9. In a large bowl, combine the cauliflower, carrots, and onion.

10. Drizzle with olive oil. Sprinkle with curry powder, cumin, turmeric, salt, and pepper. Toss to coat evenly.

11. Spread the vegetables in a single layer on the prepared baking sheet.

12. Roast in the preheated oven for 25-30 minutes, or until the vegetables are tender and lightly browned, stirring halfway through cooking.

4. Garlic Herb Roasted Vegetables

Ingredients:

- 1 small butternut squash, peeled, seeded, and cubed

- 1 large red bell pepper, seeded and sliced

- 1 yellow bell pepper, seeded and sliced

- 1 red onion, sliced

- 2 tablespoons olive oil

- 2 cloves garlic, minced

- 1 teaspoon dried thyme

- 1 teaspoon dried rosemary

- Salt and pepper, to taste

Instructions:

9. Preheat the oven to 400°F (200°C) and line a baking sheet with parchment paper.

10. In a large bowl, combine the butternut squash, bell peppers, and onion.

11. Drizzle with olive oil and sprinkle with garlic, thyme, rosemary, salt, and pepper. Toss to coat evenly.

12. Spread the vegetables in a single layer on the prepared baking sheet.

13. Roast in the preheated oven for 30-35 minutes, or until the vegetables are tender and caramelized, stirring halfway through cooking.

5. Maple Glazed Roasted Vegetables

Ingredients:

• 1 small acorn squash, peeled, seeded, and cubed

• 2 cups Brussels sprouts, trimmed and halved

• 1 sweet potato, peeled and cubed

• 2 tablespoons olive oil

• 2 tablespoons maple syrup

• 1 teaspoon cinnamon

• Salt and pepper, to taste

Instructions:

7. Preheat the oven to 400°F (200°C) and line a baking sheet with parchment paper.

8. In a large bowl, combine the acorn squash, Brussels sprouts, and sweet potato.

9. Drizzle with olive oil and maple syrup. Sprinkle with cinnamon, salt, and pepper. Toss to coat evenly.

10. Spread the vegetables in a single layer on the prepared baking sheet.

11. Roast in the preheated oven for 25-30 minutes, or until the vegetables are tender and caramelized, stirring halfway through cooking.

Quinoa and Kale Salad
1. Classic Quinoa and Kale Salad

Ingredients:

- 1 cup quinoa

- 2 cups water or vegetable broth

- 1 bunch kale, stems removed and leaves chopped

- 1/4 cup lemon juice

- 2 tablespoons olive oil

- 2 cloves garlic, minced

- 1/4 teaspoon salt

- 1/4 teaspoon black pepper

- 1/2 cup dried cranberries

- 1/2 cup chopped walnuts

Instructions:

1. Rinse quinoa under cold water and drain.

2. In a medium saucepan, combine quinoa and water or broth. Bring to a boil, then reduce heat and simmer for about 15 minutes, or until quinoa is tender and water is absorbed. Remove from heat and let cool.

3. In a large bowl, combine kale, lemon juice, olive oil, garlic, salt, and pepper. Massage the kale with your hands for a few minutes to soften it.

4. Add cooked quinoa, cranberries, and walnuts to the kale mixture. Stir until well combined.

5. Serve chilled or at room temperature.

2. Mediterranean Quinoa and Kale Salad

Ingredients:

- 1 cup quinoa
- 2 cups water or vegetable broth
- 1 bunch kale, stems removed and leaves chopped
- 1/4 cup lemon juice
- 2 tablespoons olive oil
- 2 cloves garlic, minced
- 1/2 teaspoon dried oregano
- 1/4 teaspoon salt
- 1/4 teaspoon black pepper
- 1/2 cup chopped cucumber
- 1/2 cup chopped red bell pepper
- 1/4 cup chopped red onion
- 1/4 cup crumbled feta cheese

Instructions:

1. Follow the same instructions as above to prepare the quinoa and kale.

2. In a large bowl, combine the kale, lemon juice, olive oil, garlic, oregano, salt, and pepper. Massage the kale with your hands to soften it.

3. Add the cooked quinoa, cucumber, bell pepper, red onion, and feta cheese to the bowl. Stir until well combined.

4. Serve chilled or at room temperature.

3. Asian-Inspired Quinoa and Kale Salad

Ingredients:

• 1 cup quinoa

• 2 cups water or vegetable broth

• 1 bunch kale, stems removed and leaves chopped

• 1/4 cup soy sauce or tamari

• 2 tablespoons rice vinegar

• 1 tablespoon sesame oil

• 1 tablespoon honey or maple syrup

- 1 clove garlic, minced

- 1 teaspoon grated ginger

- 1/4 cup chopped green onions

- 1/4 cup chopped cilantro

- 1/4 cup chopped peanuts or cashews

Instructions:

1. Cook the quinoa according to the package instructions. Let it cool.

2. In a large bowl, combine the kale, soy sauce, rice vinegar, sesame oil, honey or maple syrup, garlic, and ginger. Massage the kale with your hands.

3. Add the cooked quinoa, green onions, cilantro, and nuts to the bowl. Stir until well combined.

4. Serve chilled or at room temperature.

4. Apple and Cranberry Quinoa and Kale Salad

Ingredients:

- 1 cup quinoa

- 2 cups water or vegetable broth

- 1 bunch kale, stems removed and leaves chopped

- 1/4 cup apple cider vinegar

- 2 tablespoons olive oil

- 1 tablespoon honey or maple syrup

- 1/4 teaspoon salt

- 1/4 teaspoon black pepper

- 1 apple, diced

- 1/4 cup dried cranberries

- 1/4 cup chopped pecans or almonds

Instructions:

1. Cook the quinoa according to the package instructions. Let it cool.

2. In a large bowl, combine the kale, apple cider vinegar, olive oil, honey or maple syrup, salt, and pepper. Massage the kale with your hands.

3. Add the cooked quinoa, diced apple, dried cranberries, and nuts to the bowl. Stir until well combined.

4. Serve chilled or at room temperature.

5. Southwest Quinoa and Kale Salad

Ingredients:

- 1 cup quinoa

- 2 cups water or vegetable broth

- 1 bunch kale, stems removed and leaves chopped

- 1/4 cup lime juice

- 2 tablespoons olive oil

- 1 teaspoon ground cumin

- 1/2 teaspoon chili powder

- 1/4 teaspoon salt

- 1/4 teaspoon black pepper

- 1 can (15 ounces) black beans, rinsed and drained

- 1 cup corn kernels

- 1/4 cup chopped red onion

- 1/4 cup chopped fresh cilantro

- 1 avocado, diced

Instructions:

1. Cook the quinoa according to the package instructions. Let it cool.

2. In a large bowl, combine the kale, lime juice, olive oil, cumin, chili powder, salt, and pepper. Massage the kale with your hands.

3. Add the cooked quinoa, black beans, corn, red onion, cilantro, and avocado to the bowl. Stir until well combined.

4. Serve chilled or at room temperature.

Citrusy Spinach Salad

1. Classic Citrusy Spinach Salad: Ingredients:

- 4 cups baby spinach

- 1 orange, peeled and segmented

- 1/2 red onion, thinly sliced

- 1/4 cup sliced almonds

- 2 tablespoons olive oil

- 1 tablespoon balsamic vinegar

- Salt and pepper to taste

Instructions:

1. In a large bowl, combine the spinach, orange segments, red onion, and sliced almonds.

2. In a small bowl, whisk together the olive oil, balsamic vinegar, salt, and pepper.

3. Drizzle the dressing over the salad and toss to combine.

4. Serve immediately.

2. Citrusy Spinach and Strawberry Salad: Ingredients:

- 4 cups baby spinach

- 1 cup sliced strawberries

- 1/4 cup crumbled feta cheese

- 2 tablespoons sliced almonds

- 1 orange, juiced

- 2 tablespoons olive oil

- 1 teaspoon honey

- Salt and pepper to taste

Instructions:

1. In a large bowl, combine the spinach, sliced strawberries, feta cheese, and sliced almonds.

2. In a small bowl, whisk together the orange juice, olive oil, honey, salt, and pepper.

3. Drizzle the dressing over the salad and toss to combine.

4. Serve immediately.

3. Citrusy Spinach and Avocado Salad:
Ingredients:

- 4 cups baby spinach

- 1 avocado, diced

- 1/4 cup sliced red onion

- 2 tablespoons chopped fresh cilantro

- 1 orange, peeled and segmented

- 2 tablespoons olive oil

- 1 tablespoon lime juice

- Salt and pepper to taste

Instructions:

1. In a large bowl, combine the spinach, diced avocado, sliced red onion, chopped cilantro, and orange segments.

2. In a small bowl, whisk together the olive oil, lime juice, salt, and pepper.

3. Drizzle the dressing over the salad and toss to combine.

4. Serve immediately.

4. Citrusy Spinach and Chickpea Salad: Ingredients:

- 4 cups baby spinach

- 1 can (15 ounces) chickpeas, rinsed and drained

- 1/2 cup diced red bell pepper

- 1/4 cup chopped fresh parsley

- 1 orange, juiced

- 2 tablespoons olive oil

- 1 teaspoon ground cumin

- Salt and pepper to taste

Instructions:

1. In a large bowl, combine the spinach, chickpeas, diced red bell pepper, and chopped parsley.

2. In a small bowl, whisk together the orange juice, olive oil, ground cumin, salt, and pepper.

3. Drizzle the dressing over the salad and toss to combine.

4. Serve immediately.

5. Citrusy Spinach and Quinoa Salad: Ingredients:

- 2 cups cooked quinoa

- 4 cups baby spinach

- 1/2 cup dried cranberries

- 1/4 cup chopped pecans

- 1 orange, juiced

- 2 tablespoons olive oil

- 1 tablespoon maple syrup

- Salt and pepper to taste

Instructions:

1. In a large bowl, combine the cooked quinoa, spinach, dried cranberries, and chopped pecans.

2. In a small bowl, whisk together the orange juice, olive oil, maple syrup, salt, and pepper.

3. Drizzle the dressing over the salad and toss to combine.

4. Serve immediately.

Chapter 3: Wholesome Main Courses

Lemon Garlic Salmon

1. Lemon Garlic Herb Salmon

Ingredients:

• 4 salmon fillets

• 4 cloves garlic, minced

• 2 tablespoons olive oil

• 2 tablespoons fresh lemon juice

• 1 tablespoon chopped fresh parsley

• Salt and pepper to taste

Instructions:

1. Preheat the oven to 375°F (190°C).

2. In a small bowl, combine the minced garlic, olive oil, lemon juice, parsley, salt, and pepper.

3. Place the salmon fillets on a baking sheet lined with parchment paper.

4. Spoon the garlic mixture over the salmon fillets, spreading it evenly.

5. Bake in the preheated oven for 12-15 minutes, or until the salmon is cooked through and flakes easily with a fork.

2. Lemon Garlic Butter Salmon

Ingredients:

• 4 salmon fillets

• 4 cloves garlic, minced

• 4 tablespoons unsalted butter, melted

• 2 tablespoons fresh lemon juice

• 1 teaspoon lemon zest

• Salt and pepper to taste

Instructions:

1. Preheat the oven to 375°F (190°C).

2. In a small bowl, combine the minced garlic, melted butter, lemon juice, lemon zest, salt, and pepper.

3. Place the salmon fillets on a baking sheet lined with parchment paper.

4. Spoon the garlic butter mixture over the salmon fillets, spreading it evenly.

5. Bake in the preheated oven for 12-15 minutes, or until the salmon is cooked through and flakes easily with a fork.

3. Lemon Garlic Dijon Salmon

Ingredients:

• 4 salmon fillets

• 4 cloves garlic, minced

• 2 tablespoons olive oil

• 2 tablespoons fresh lemon juice

• 2 tablespoons Dijon mustard

• Salt and pepper to taste

Instructions:

1. Preheat the oven to 375°F (190°C).

2. In a small bowl, combine the minced garlic, olive oil, lemon juice, Dijon mustard, salt, and pepper.

3. Place the salmon fillets on a baking sheet lined with parchment paper.

4. Spoon the garlic Dijon mixture over the salmon fillets, spreading it evenly.

5. Bake in the preheated oven for 12-15 minutes, or until the salmon is cooked through and flakes easily with a fork.

4. Lemon Garlic Honey Salmon

Ingredients:

• 4 salmon fillets

• 4 cloves garlic, minced

• 2 tablespoons olive oil

• 2 tablespoons fresh lemon juice

• 2 tablespoons honey

• Salt and pepper to taste

Instructions:

1. Preheat the oven to 375°F (190°C).

2. In a small bowl, combine the minced garlic, olive oil, lemon juice, honey, salt, and pepper.

3. Place the salmon fillets on a baking sheet lined with parchment paper.

4. Spoon the garlic honey mixture over the salmon fillets, spreading it evenly.

5. Bake in the preheated oven for 12-15 minutes, or until the salmon is cooked through and flakes easily with a fork.

5. Lemon Garlic Pesto Salmon

Ingredients:

• 4 salmon fillets

• 4 cloves garlic, minced

• 2 tablespoons olive oil

• 2 tablespoons fresh lemon juice

• 4 tablespoons pesto sauce

• Salt and pepper to taste

Instructions:

1. Preheat the oven to 375°F (190°C).

2. In a small bowl, combine the minced garlic, olive oil, lemon juice, pesto sauce, salt, and pepper.

3. Place the salmon fillets on a baking sheet lined with parchment paper.

4. Spoon the garlic pesto mixture over the salmon fillets, spreading it evenly.

5. Bake in the preheated oven for 12-15 minutes, or until the salmon is cooked through and flakes easily with a fork.

Lentil and Sweet Potato Curry

Certainly! Here are five variations of Lentil and Sweet Potato Curry, each with a unique twist:

1. Classic Lentil and Sweet Potato Curry

Ingredients:

• 1 cup dried lentils, rinsed and drained

- 2 medium sweet potatoes, peeled and diced

- 1 onion, chopped

- 2 cloves garlic, minced

- 1 tablespoon curry powder

- 1 teaspoon ground cumin

- 1 teaspoon ground turmeric

- 1 can (14 ounces) diced tomatoes

- 1 can (14 ounces) coconut milk

- Salt and pepper, to taste

- Fresh cilantro, for garnish

- Cooked rice, for serving

Instructions:

1. In a large pot, heat oil over medium heat. Add the onion and garlic, and cook until softened.

2. Stir in the curry powder, cumin, and turmeric, and cook for another minute.

3. Add the lentils, sweet potatoes, diced tomatoes (with juices), and coconut milk. Bring to a boil.

4. Reduce heat, cover, and simmer for about 25-30 minutes, or until lentils and sweet potatoes are tender.

5. Season with salt and pepper to taste. Serve over cooked rice and garnish with fresh cilantro.

2. Spicy Lentil and Sweet Potato Curry

Ingredients:

• Same as the classic recipe, but add:

• 1-2 teaspoons red pepper flakes (adjust to taste)

• 1 teaspoon paprika

• 1 teaspoon garam masala

• 1 tablespoon sriracha sauce (optional, for extra heat)

Instructions:

• Follow the same instructions as the classic recipe, adding the extra spices and sriracha sauce when adding the lentils and sweet potatoes.

3. Coconut Lentil and Sweet Potato Curry

Ingredients:

• Same as the classic recipe, but replace the diced tomatoes with 1 can (14 ounces) of tomato sauce and add:

• 1/2 cup shredded coconut (unsweetened)

Instructions:

• Follow the same instructions as the classic recipe, using tomato sauce instead of diced tomatoes and adding shredded coconut with the lentils and sweet potatoes.

4. Peanut Lentil and Sweet Potato Curry

Ingredients:

• Same as the classic recipe, but add:

• 1/2 cup creamy peanut butter

• 1 tablespoon soy sauce

• 1 teaspoon ground ginger

• Crushed peanuts, for garnish

Instructions:

• Follow the same instructions as the classic recipe, adding the peanut butter, soy sauce, and ground ginger when adding the lentils and sweet potatoes. Serve garnished with crushed peanuts.

5. Spinach Lentil and Sweet Potato Curry

Ingredients:

• Same as the classic recipe, but add:

• 4 cups fresh spinach leaves, chopped

• 1 can (14 ounces) chickpeas, drained and rinsed

Instructions:

• Follow the same instructions as the classic recipe, adding the spinach and chickpeas when the lentils and sweet potatoes are almost tender. Cook for an additional 5-10 minutes, or until spinach is wilted.

Chapter 4: Satisfying Sides

Garlic Mashed Cauliflower

1. Classic Garlic Mashed Cauliflower

Ingredients:

- 1 head of cauliflower, chopped into florets

- 2-3 cloves of garlic, minced

- 2 tablespoons of butter

- Salt and pepper, to taste

- Fresh chives, chopped (optional, for garnish)

Instructions:

1. Steam or boil the cauliflower until very tender.

2. In a skillet, melt the butter over medium heat. Add the minced garlic and sauté for 1-2 minutes, until fragrant.

3. Transfer the cooked cauliflower to a food processor. Add the garlic-butter mixture, salt, and pepper.

4. Blend until smooth and creamy.

5. Adjust seasoning if needed. Garnish with chopped chives before serving.

2. Parmesan Garlic Mashed Cauliflower

Ingredients:

• 1 head of cauliflower, chopped into florets

• 2-3 cloves of garlic, minced

• 2 tablespoons of butter

• 1/4 cup of grated Parmesan cheese

• Salt and pepper, to taste

• Fresh parsley, chopped (optional, for garnish)

Instructions:

1. Prepare the cauliflower as in the previous recipe.

2. In a skillet, melt the butter over medium heat. Add the minced garlic and sauté for 1-2 minutes.

3. Blend the cooked cauliflower with the garlic-butter mixture, Parmesan cheese, salt, and pepper until smooth.

4. Adjust seasoning if needed. Garnish with chopped parsley before serving.

3. Roasted Garlic Mashed Cauliflower

Ingredients:

• 1 head of cauliflower, chopped into florets

• 1 whole garlic bulb

• Olive oil

• Salt and pepper, to taste

• 2 tablespoons of butter

• Fresh thyme leaves, chopped (optional, for garnish)

Instructions:

1. Roast the cauliflower florets and whole garlic bulb in the oven at 400°F (200°C) for about 25-30 minutes, or until tender and slightly caramelized.

2. Squeeze the roasted garlic cloves out of the bulb and mash them with a fork.

3. Blend the roasted cauliflower, mashed garlic, butter, salt, and pepper until smooth.

4. Adjust seasoning if needed. Garnish with chopped thyme leaves before serving.

4. Herbed Garlic Mashed Cauliflower

Ingredients:

• 1 head of cauliflower, chopped into florets

• 2-3 cloves of garlic, minced

• 2 tablespoons of butter

• 1/4 cup of chopped fresh herbs (such as parsley, chives, and thyme)

• Salt and pepper, to taste

Instructions:

1. Prepare the cauliflower as in the first recipe.

2. In a skillet, melt the butter over medium heat. Add the minced garlic and sauté for 1-2 minutes.

3. Blend the cooked cauliflower with the garlic-butter mixture, chopped herbs, salt, and pepper until smooth.

4. Adjust seasoning if needed. Serve garnished with additional chopped herbs.

5. Spicy Garlic Mashed Cauliflower

Ingredients:

• 1 head of cauliflower, chopped into florets

• 2-3 cloves of garlic, minced

• 2 tablespoons of butter

• 1/2 teaspoon of red pepper flakes (adjust to taste)

• Salt and pepper, to taste

• Fresh cilantro, chopped (optional, for garnish)

Instructions:

1. Prepare the cauliflower as in the first recipe.

2. In a skillet, melt the butter over medium heat. Add the minced garlic and red pepper flakes and sauté for 1-2 minutes.

3. Blend the cooked cauliflower with the garlic-butter mixture, salt, and pepper until smooth.

4. Adjust seasoning if needed. Garnish with chopped cilantro before serving.

Roasted Brussels Sprouts

1. Classic Roasted Brussels Sprouts

Ingredients:

• 1 pound Brussels sprouts, trimmed and halved

• 2 tablespoons olive oil

• Salt and pepper, to taste

Instructions:

1. Preheat the oven to 400°F (200°C).

2. In a large bowl, toss the Brussels sprouts with olive oil, salt, and pepper until evenly coated.

3. Spread the Brussels sprouts in a single layer on a baking sheet.

4. Roast in the preheated oven for 25-30 minutes, or until the Brussels sprouts are tender and caramelized, stirring halfway through cooking.

2. Balsamic Glazed Brussels Sprouts

Ingredients:

• 1 pound Brussels sprouts, trimmed and halved

• 2 tablespoons olive oil

• 2 tablespoons balsamic vinegar

• 1 tablespoon honey

• Salt and pepper, to taste

Instructions:

1. Preheat the oven to 400°F (200°C).

2. In a large bowl, toss the Brussels sprouts with olive oil, salt, and pepper until evenly coated.

3. Spread the Brussels sprouts in a single layer on a baking sheet.

4. Roast in the preheated oven for 20-25 minutes, or until the Brussels sprouts are tender, stirring halfway through cooking.

5. In a small saucepan, combine balsamic vinegar and honey. Cook over medium heat until the mixture is reduced and thickened, about 5 minutes.

6. Drizzle the balsamic glaze over the roasted Brussels sprouts before serving.

3. Parmesan Roasted Brussels Sprouts

Ingredients:

• 1 pound Brussels sprouts, trimmed and halved

• 2 tablespoons olive oil

• 1/4 cup grated Parmesan cheese

• Salt and pepper, to taste

Instructions:

1. Preheat the oven to 400°F (200°C).

2. In a large bowl, toss the Brussels sprouts with olive oil, salt, and pepper until evenly coated.

3. Spread the Brussels sprouts in a single layer on a baking sheet.

4. Roast in the preheated oven for 20-25 minutes, or until the Brussels sprouts are tender and lightly browned, stirring halfway through cooking.

5. Sprinkle the roasted Brussels sprouts with Parmesan cheese before serving.

4. Garlic Roasted Brussels Sprouts

Ingredients:

• 1 pound Brussels sprouts, trimmed and halved

• 3 tablespoons olive oil

• 3 cloves garlic, minced

• Salt and pepper, to taste

Instructions:

1. Preheat the oven to 400°F (200°C).

2. In a large bowl, toss the Brussels sprouts with olive oil, minced garlic, salt, and pepper until evenly coated.

3. Spread the Brussels sprouts in a single layer on a baking sheet.

4. Roast in the preheated oven for 20-25 minutes, or until the Brussels sprouts are tender and caramelized, stirring halfway through cooking.

5. Maple Dijon Roasted Brussels Sprouts

Ingredients:

• 1 pound Brussels sprouts, trimmed and halved

• 2 tablespoons olive oil

• 2 tablespoons maple syrup

• 1 tablespoon Dijon mustard

• Salt and pepper, to taste

Instructions:

1. Preheat the oven to 400°F (200°C).

2. In a large bowl, whisk together olive oil, maple syrup, Dijon mustard, salt, and pepper.

3. Add the Brussels sprouts to the bowl and toss until evenly coated.

4. Spread the Brussels sprouts in a single layer on a baking sheet.

5. Roast in the preheated oven for 20-25 minutes, or until the Brussels sprouts are tender and caramelized, stirring halfway through cooking.

Chapter 5: Decadent Desserts

Avocado Chocolate Mousse

1. Classic Avocado Chocolate Mousse:
Ingredients:

• 2 ripe avocados

• 1/4 cup cocoa powder

• 1/4 cup maple syrup or honey

• 1/2 teaspoon vanilla extract

• Pinch of salt

• Optional toppings: shaved chocolate, berries, whipped cream

Instructions:

1. Cut the avocados in half, remove the pits, and scoop the flesh into a blender or food processor.

2. Add the cocoa powder, maple syrup or honey, vanilla extract, and a pinch of salt.

3. Blend until smooth and creamy, scraping down the sides as needed.

4. Spoon the mousse into serving dishes and refrigerate for at least 30 minutes.

5. Serve with your favorite toppings, such as shaved chocolate, berries, or whipped cream.

2. Mint Chocolate Avocado Mousse: Ingredients:

• 2 ripe avocados

• 1/4 cup cocoa powder

• 1/4 cup maple syrup or honey

• 1/2 teaspoon peppermint extract

• Pinch of salt

• Optional toppings: chocolate chips, fresh mint leaves

Instructions:

1. Follow the same instructions as the Classic Avocado Chocolate Mousse, but add 1/2 teaspoon of peppermint extract to the blender along with the other ingredients.

2. Blend until smooth and creamy.

3. Refrigerate, then serve with chocolate chips and fresh mint leaves as toppings.

3. Coconut Avocado Chocolate Mousse:
Ingredients:

• 2 ripe avocados

• 1/4 cup cocoa powder

• 1/4 cup coconut milk

• 1/4 cup maple syrup or honey

• 1/2 teaspoon vanilla extract

• Pinch of salt

• Optional toppings: toasted coconut flakes, sliced almonds

Instructions:

1. Blend all ingredients in a blender or food processor until smooth and creamy.

2. Refrigerate for at least 30 minutes.

3. Serve with toasted coconut flakes and sliced almonds on top.

4. Almond Butter Avocado Chocolate Mousse: Ingredients:

• 2 ripe avocados

• 1/4 cup cocoa powder

• 1/4 cup almond butter

• 1/4 cup maple syrup or honey

• 1/2 teaspoon vanilla extract

• Pinch of salt

• Optional toppings: sliced almonds, chocolate syrup

Instructions:

1. Blend all ingredients in a blender or food processor until smooth.

2. Refrigerate for at least 30 minutes.

3. Serve with sliced almonds and a drizzle of chocolate syrup on top.

5. Raspberry Swirl Avocado Chocolate Mousse: Ingredients:

- 2 ripe avocados

- 1/4 cup cocoa powder

- 1/4 cup maple syrup or honey

- 1/2 teaspoon vanilla extract

- Pinch of salt

- 1/4 cup fresh or frozen raspberries, thawed

- Optional toppings: fresh raspberries, chocolate curls

Instructions:

1. Blend the avocados, cocoa powder, maple syrup or honey, vanilla extract, and salt until smooth.

2. Spoon the mousse into serving dishes.

3. In a separate bowl, mash the raspberries with a fork until smooth.

4. Swirl the raspberry puree into the mousse.

5. Refrigerate for at least 30 minutes.

6. Serve with fresh raspberries and chocolate curls on top.

1. Classic Vanilla Chia Seed Pudding

Ingredients:

• 1/4 cup chia seeds

• 1 cup almond milk (or any other milk of choice)

• 1 tablespoon maple syrup (or sweetener of choice)

• 1/2 teaspoon vanilla extract

Instructions:

1. In a bowl, mix chia seeds, almond milk, maple syrup, and vanilla extract.

2. Stir well to combine.

3. Cover and refrigerate for at least 4 hours or overnight.

4. Stir well before serving. Add toppings like fresh berries or nuts if desired.

2. Chocolate Chia Seed Pudding

Ingredients:

- 1/4 cup chia seeds

- 1 cup almond milk (or any other milk of choice)

- 1 tablespoon cocoa powder

- 1 tablespoon maple syrup (or sweetener of choice)

Instructions:

1. In a bowl, mix chia seeds, almond milk, cocoa powder, and maple syrup.

2. Stir well to combine.

3. Cover and refrigerate for at least 4 hours or overnight.

4. Stir well before serving. Add toppings like sliced bananas or shredded coconut if desired.

3. Strawberry Chia Seed Pudding

Ingredients:

- 1/4 cup chia seeds

- 1 cup almond milk (or any other milk of choice)

- 1/2 cup mashed strawberries

- 1 tablespoon honey (or sweetener of choice)

Instructions:

1. In a bowl, mix chia seeds, almond milk, mashed strawberries, and honey.

2. Stir well to combine.

3. Cover and refrigerate for at least 4 hours or overnight.

4. Stir well before serving. Top with additional sliced strawberries if desired.

4. Peanut Butter Banana Chia Seed Pudding

Ingredients:

- 1/4 cup chia seeds

- 1 cup almond milk (or any other milk of choice)

- 1 ripe banana, mashed

- 2 tablespoons peanut butter

- 1 tablespoon honey (or sweetener of choice)

Instructions:

1. In a bowl, mix chia seeds, almond milk, mashed banana, peanut butter, and honey.

2. Stir well to combine.

3. Cover and refrigerate for at least 4 hours or overnight.

4. Stir well before serving. Top with a drizzle of melted peanut butter if desired.

5. Coconut Mango Chia Seed Pudding

Ingredients:

- 1/4 cup chia seeds

- 1 cup coconut milk

- 1/2 cup diced mango

- 1 tablespoon honey (or sweetener of choice)

- 2 tablespoons shredded coconut

Instructions:

1. In a bowl, mix chia seeds, coconut milk, diced mango, honey, and shredded coconut.

2. Stir well to combine.

3. Cover and refrigerate for at least 4 hours or overnight.

4. Stir well before serving. Top with additional diced mango and shredded coconut if desired.

Enjoy these delicious and nutritious Chia Seed Pudding recipe

Conclusion

In conclusion, managing Graves' disease involves a comprehensive approach that includes medical treatment, lifestyle modifications, and dietary changes. While diet alone cannot cure the condition, it can play a significant role in alleviating symptoms, supporting thyroid function, and promoting overall health.

A diet for Graves' disease should focus on consuming nutrient-dense foods, limiting iodine-rich foods, managing goitrogenic foods, and staying well-hydrated. It's important to work closely with healthcare providers or dietitians to develop a personalized diet plan that meets individual needs and complements medical treatment.

By adopting a balanced and mindful approach to diet and lifestyle, individuals with Graves' disease can better manage their condition, reduce symptoms, and improve their quality of life.

Made in the USA
Las Vegas, NV
19 June 2024

91213969R00046